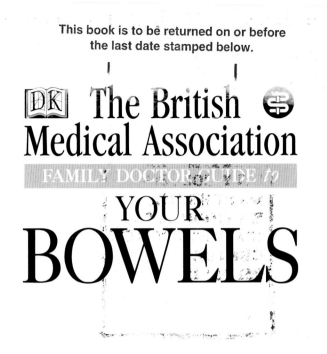

DK The British
Medical Association
FAMILY DOCTOR GUIDE to
YOUR
BOWELS

The British Medical Association

FAMILY DOCTOR GUIDE to

YOUR
BOWELS

DR. KEN HEATON

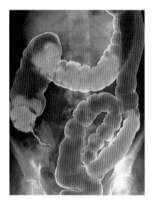

MEDICAL EDITOR
DR. TONY SMITH

DORLING KINDERSLEY
LONDON • NEW YORK • SYDNEY • MOSCOW
www.dk.com

IMPORTANT

This book is not designed as a substitute for personal medical advice but as a supplement to that advice for the patient who wishes to understand more about his/her condition.

Before taking any form of treatment **YOU SHOULD ALWAYS CONSULT YOUR MEDICAL PRACTITIONER.**

In particular (without limit) you should note that advances in medical science occur rapidly and some of the information contained in this book about drugs and treatment may very soon be out of date.

PLEASE NOTE

The author regrets that he cannot enter into any correspondence with readers.

A DORLING KINDERSLEY BOOK
www.dk.com

Senior Editor Mary Lindsay
Senior Designer Sarah Hall
Project Editor David Tombesi-Walton
Designer Laura Watson
DTP Designer Jason Little
Production Controller Michelle Thomas

Managing Editor Stephanie Jackson
Managing Art Editor Nigel Duffield

Produced for Dorling Kindersley Limited by
Design Revolution, Queens Park Villa,
30 West Drive, Brighton, East Sussex BN2 2GE.
Editorial Manager Ian Whitelaw
Art Director Fiona Roberts
Editor Julie Whitaker
Designer Vanessa Good

Published in Great Britain in 1999 by
Dorling Kindersley Limited,
9 Henrietta Street, London WC2E 8PS2

2 4 6 8 10 9 7 5 3 1

A CIP catalogue record for this book is available from the British Library

ISBN 0 7513 0677 0

Reproduced by Colourscan, Singapore
Printed in Hong Kong by Wing King Tong

Contents

Introduction

Although bowel complaints are extremely common (1 in 5 people suffer from some kind of disorder at any one time), we are conditioned to keep any health worries about our intestines to ourselves. Our language reflects this reluctance – we may say we are going to the toilet, but we are unable to discuss what happens there.

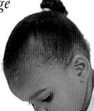

EARLY LEARNING
Children should learn from an early age that bowel movements are a normal part of life.

A TABOO SUBJECT

Have you ever wondered why bowel movements and stools are taboo subjects? There are many reasons for this. From earliest childhood we are all conditioned to regard stools as dirty, disgusting and maybe even dangerous. The nasty things must be disposed of as quickly as possible. The act of passing stools is an unfortunate necessity and an entirely private matter. As for the organs which produce stools, most of us prefer not to think about them and, if we do, we regard them as mysterious, unpredictable and rather disgraceful.

There are grounds for some of these beliefs and attitudes. Stools are usually smelly – sometimes appallingly so. Diseases can be spread from people's stools to other people. The act of opening the bowels is an undignified affair, best done in private, and sometimes it is uncomfortable. The colon and rectum (which make stools) are extremely mysterious organs – perhaps the least understood organs in the body. And who amongst us has not been embarrassed by passing wind in company?

Distaste and reticence, however, can go too far. Stools and wind do not have to be smelly – odour depends to some extent on what we eat. Stools cause the spread of disease only when people are careless about washing their hands or when sewage gets into our water supplies.

Opening the bowels need not be uncomfortable. Our knowledge of the bowels has increased enormously in recent years, and doctors can now actually diagnose and cure or relieve nearly all the disorders of the bowels.

Disorders of the bowels are extremely common. In fact, most people suffer from problems with bowel function or piles (haemorrhoids), or both, at some time in their lives. At any given time, one in five of the population is experiencing discomfort from their bowels, and one in 40 of us will develop cancer in the bowel, which can largely be prevented by eating the right food.

The food we eat and the way we live our lives have enormous effects on our bowels. This book tries to explain all these matters: it will help you to keep the workings of your bowels comfortable and it will tell you what to do if things go wrong. Medical terms are explained in the Glossary (see pp.82–83).

A PRIVATE AFFAIR
Only the young feel comfortable opening their bowels in public. We soon learn that such an activity is best done in total privacy.

Disorders Caused by Colonic Bacteria

Most of the bacteria that live in the colon are harmless, but when combined with other factors, for example bad hygiene practices or a poor diet, they may contribute to the onset of disease.

INFECTIONS WITHIN THE BOWELS
When, through bad hygiene, one person's colonic bacteria get into another person's food or drink, they can cause attacks of gastroenteritis and diarrhoea.

E.COLI BACTERIA
These bacteria (magnified here 5,000 times) exist harmlessly in the colons of humans and animals. They are, however, sometimes responsible for food poisoning.

INFECTIONS OUTSIDE THE BOWELS
When, through injury or disease, the bacteria get into other parts of the body they can produce dangerous infections such as cystitis.

NON-INFECTIOUS DISEASES
Some of the chemical substances released by colonic bacteria may cause disease, especially cancer of the bowel and gallstones. However, this may only be a problem when a high-calorie, low-fibre diet is eaten.

9

SOME WORDS AND PHRASES

The word 'bowels' is one of those vague words that can mean different things at different times. Sometimes it is used to describe both the large and the small intestines, but often use of the term is limited to the large intestine or colon, which is the last part of the alimentary canal, or digestive tube.

When people speak of 'using the bowels', 'emptying the bowels', 'moving the bowels', or 'opening the bowels' they are trying to speak politely of that unmentionable activity which is correctly called defecation. A less technical way of saying the same thing is 'passing a stool'. Stools, faeces and bowel motions all mean the same thing to doctors. It is strange that these words are rarely used in polite conversation; most people use roundabout expressions instead.

Gas passed from the rectum (back passage) is properly called flatus. Many people refer to it as wind or flatulence, but this is confusing because other people use the terms wind and flatulence to mean belching (burping) or to mean bloated feelings or gurglings from the abdomen.

'Fart' has the advantage of meaning only one thing, but this term is even less acceptable in polite conversation than faeces. Probably the nearest we have to an expression which is both unambiguous and reasonably polite is 'voiding wind'.

GOOD HYGIENE
Persuade young children to wash their hands after using the toilet, and they should keep the habit for life.

KEY POINTS

- We are conditioned from an early age to regard stools as dirty, disgusting and even dangerous.
- Disorders of the bowel are extremely common: at any moment in time 1 in 5 of the population is experiencing bowel discomfort.
- The food we eat and the way we live our lives have enormous effects on our bowels.

A brief guide to the bowel

The digestive tract or tube consists of the stomach, large and small intestines, the colon, rectum and anal canal. The colon begins just above the right groin where it is known as the caecum and from which springs the appendix. It continues as the ascending colon, which climbs to just below the ribs on the right of the body, and then swings across to the opposite side as the transverse colon.

With a second sharp bend it turns downward as the descending colon, and finally makes a curious loop known as the sigmoid (named after the squiggly Greek letter sigma or Σ) before joining on to the rectum. The word rectum comes from the Latin word for straight, which is odd because actually it bends sharply backwards just before it joins on to the anal canal. It does straighten out, however, while the bowels are being opened, when it functions simply as a tube conducting stools from the sigmoid colon to the outside world. Strictly speaking it is

THE DIGESTIVE SYSTEM
The digestive system lies between the rib cage and the pubic bone. It digests food so that the body absorbs nutrients and eliminates waste.

The Large and Small Intestines

The intestines form the major part of the digestive system. The small intestine absorbs nutrients from food as it passes down its length. The large intestine ferments any undigested food and extracts water from its contents so that they turn from liquid to solid, ready to be expelled as faeces.

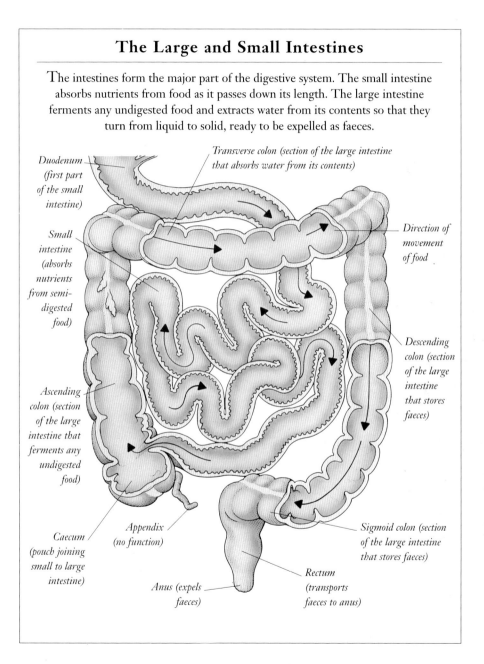

Duodenum (first part of the small intestine)

Transverse colon (section of the large intestine that absorbs water from its contents)

Small intestine (absorbs nutrients from semi-digested food)

Direction of movement of food

Descending colon (section of the large intestine that stores faeces)

Ascending colon (section of the large intestine that ferments any undigested food)

Caecum (pouch joining small to large intestine)

Appendix (no function)

Anus (expels faeces)

Rectum (transports faeces to anus)

Sigmoid colon (section of the large intestine that stores faeces)

the anal canal that does the last part of this job, but the canal is only an inch or so long and is really just a device for keeping stools and gas inside their owner until he or she decides to let them out.

The anal canal is the only part of the alimentary tube after the throat over which we exert conscious control. The gut is a muscular tube, but the throat and the anal canal are the only parts of the tube whose muscle fibres are of the same kind as the muscles in our arms and legs. The anal muscle fibres are arranged as a two-part closing system. First, there is a sling of fibres round the upper end of the tube. When this muscle contracts it exerts a forward pull and so maintains the sharp angle where the rectum joins the anus; at the same time it presses the front and back of the canal against each other. Second, there is a ring of fibres whose contraction makes the hole in the tube narrower. Both sets of fibres are contracting gently all the time without any conscious effort on our part (just like many other muscles in the body). We have to relax these muscles in order to be able to pass a stool or some wind.

THE LINING OF THE BOWEL

Between the muscular wall and the interior of the bowel (the lumen) there is an all-important lining. In the anal canal this lining is simply skin, but under it are clumps of soft, spongy material called the anal cushions. In the rest of the bowel the lining is a delicate mucous membrane or mucosa. This fragile lining has the difficult task of being a barrier to dangerous things like bacteria and viruses, while at the same time letting through into the bloodstream the good things like water and salts which we cannot afford to lose in the stools. It is a balancing act.

If the mucosa absorbs too much water, the stools become hard and difficult to pass; if it absorbs too little, they are liquid and copious and the anal muscles have difficulty keeping them in. At one extreme there is constipation, at the other diarrhoea and incontinence.

MOVEMENTS OF THE BOWEL

The muscles of the bowel seldom rest – every few seconds they contract briefly in short sections of bowel. These contractions make the bowel narrower and drive

---

Movement through the Bowel

Different types of muscle contraction move waste products through the colon. Type 1 moves the contents around within the intestine without moving them forwards. Type 2 propels the contents down towards the rectum for defecation.

Shuttle contractions move the contents back and forth

Peristaltic contractions propel the contents through the large intestine towards the rectum

A mass movement squeezes faeces into the sigmoid colon and then into the rectum

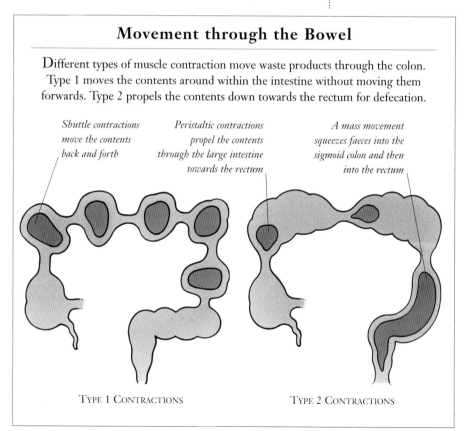

TYPE 1 CONTRACTIONS   TYPE 2 CONTRACTIONS

its contents into neighbouring sections that are relaxed. Most of these movements simply shuttle the contents back and forth, presumably to increase their exposure to the mucosa and so ensure the maximum absorption of valuable water and salts. Now and again a wave of contraction passes round the entire colon, pushing its contents forwards. This is known as mass peristalsis and it occurs mostly at meal times, especially during breakfast. This explains why many people feel the need to open their bowels after breakfast. In others, mass peristalsis is set off by getting out of bed and dressing.

RECOGNISING SENSATIONS

The fortunate among us experience sensations from our bowel only when we need to pass stools and wind. Both sensations are signals from the rectum saying it is receiving material from the sigmoid and the amazing thing is that we can tell whether the material is solid, liquid or gaseous. The distinction is probably made by miniature sensors at the top end of the anal canal. Many people also feel wriggling movements in their abdomen when gas is moved from one part of the colon to another. At the same time, a gurgling sound may be heard. Other people feel a wave of discomfort, which may even be painful, when the need to open the bowels is strong, for example, if the stool is looser than usual. All these sensations are perfectly normal, up to a point.

Discomfort and pain from the colon are extremely common in otherwise healthy people (see Irritable Bowel Syndrome, pp.56–62). Sometimes this implies that the bowel is contracting strongly, but it often means that the bowel has become more sensitive or the person has become more aware of their bowel for some reason.

BACTERIA: FRIENDS AND FOES

A unique feature of the large intestine is that it is host to a huge number of bacteria. This is not as alarming as it sounds because the bacteria present in the large intestine are nearly all harmless. Some animals – the herbivores other than ruminants – actually depend for their lives on the bacteria in their intestines; the grass they eat is useless until it has been fermented by the bacteria.

We humans do not need our bacteria for any vital function, but neither do we need to fear them despite their vast numbers. They are scavengers, living off the undigested remnants of our food and the mucus and dead cells that are constantly shed by the lining of the colon. They are also responsible for the gas (flatus) that we pass from the rectum.

Laboratory experiments show that if animals do not have bacteria in their guts they are more prone to disease – germ-free animals are fragile creatures. The chances are that the same would be true of humans, so by all means respect your bowel bacteria but do not live in fear of them.

RELYING ON BACTERIA
Herbivores such as horses and deer rely on the action of bacteria in their intestines to perform an essential part of digestion.

WHAT IS NORMAL?

The large bowel and its products have never been popular subjects for research so, perhaps unsurprisingly, scientific data on them are limited.

However, thanks to recent scientific research, we now have the following facts and figures about the adult British population.

Most people claim to open their bowels once a day but, when they are asked to record all their bowel openings, it turns out that a regular 24-hour cycle is present in only 40 per cent of men and 33 per cent of women, and a twice or three times a day habit in another seven per cent and four per cent respectively. So most people are irregular in their habits. This is especially true of younger women. About 10 per cent of women and about three per cent of men go only two or three times a week, while one in a hundred women go only once a week or even less often.

It is hard to state what is normal and what is abnormal. Some doctors consider that any bowel habit is normal so long as it causes no discomfort. However, if the bowels open only two or three times a week it is likely that the passage of food residues through the colon is so slow that, in time, there will be repercussions on general health. Unfortunately, a once-daily habit is no guarantee that everything is right. It is possible to go once a day but every time be four or five days late! A better guide to how long a stool has been in the colon is the appearance of the stool, rather than frequency of motion.

Stools have been classified into seven types, on what is called the Bristol Stool Form Scale (see opposite), according to their appearance as seen in the toilet water. Type 1 has spent the longest in the colon and Type 7 the least time.

Stools at the lumpy end of the scale are hard to pass and often require a lot of straining. Stools at the loose or liquid end of the spectrum can be too easy to pass – the need to pass them is urgent and accidents can happen. The ideal stools are Types 3 and 4, especially Type 4, as they are most likely to glide out without any

The Bristol Stool Form Scale

This chart lists the range of stool types most commonly passed. Ideally you should be aiming for a Type 4 stool.

TYPE 1	Separate hard lumps, like nuts
TYPE 2	Sausage-like but lumpy
TYPE 3	Like a sausage but with cracks in the surface
TYPE 4	Like a sausage or snake, smooth and soft
TYPE 5	Soft blobs with clear-cut edges
TYPE 6	Fluffy pieces with ragged edges, a mushy stool
TYPE 7	Watery, no solid pieces

fuss whatsoever. Also, they are least likely to leave you with an annoying feeling that something is left behind.

The average passage time of undigested food residues through the human gut is about 50 hours in men and 57 hours in women, but ranges from well under 20 to over 100 hours. It also changes from one day to the next. Most of this time is spent in the colon.

The average weight of a stool is about 100 g (3.5 oz) but, again, this varies a lot. The colour of normal stools is always brown, but, curiously, the nature of the brown pigments is unknown. The average stool is 75 per cent water, but most of this water is locked up inside bacteria and undigested plant cells. Half to two-thirds of the stool

The Ideal Bowel Movement

The features listed here are all likely to accompany the passing of a type 4 stool (see the Bristol Stool Form Scale, p. 19).

- The feeling you need to go is definite but not irresistible
- Once you sit down on the loo there is no delay
- No conscious effort or straining is needed
- The stool glides out smoothly and comfortably
- Afterwards there is only a pleasant feeling of relief

is bacteria – some living, some dead – and the rest consists mainly of the undigested residues of plant foods (dietary fibre). Thanks to bacterial activity, there are hundreds of different organic compounds in stools, mainly present in trace amounts.

The average person is said to void wind 12 times in 24 hours. This fact was established in young men (American students) and the situation may be different in older people and in women. There is much person-to-person variation.

The lack of basic scientific data in this field of human experience is extraordinary. For example, we do not know how many stools float in water and how many sink, nor how long people spend over the act of defecation. It is widely taught that straining (holding the breath and pushing) is a normal and necessary part of defecation. However, recent research has shown that straining is a minority practice and, what's more, depends on the type, size and consistency of the stool. The most difficult stools to pass are small ones and the broad, lumpy ones. In practice, these are Types 1 and 2, or occasionally 3.

Progress of Food through the Digestive System

After swallowing, food moves by muscular contractions through the digestive system. The time spent in each area depends on the stage of digestion. Duration also varies with food type and quantity, and on an individual and daily basis.

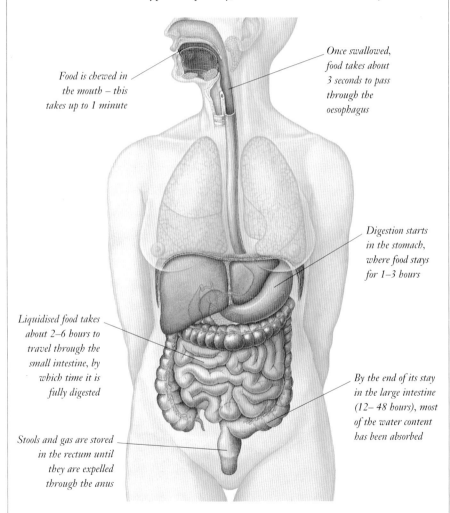

Food is chewed in the mouth – this takes up to 1 minute

Once swallowed, food takes about 3 seconds to pass through the oesophagus

Digestion starts in the stomach, where food stays for 1–3 hours

Liquidised food takes about 2–6 hours to travel through the small intestine, by which time it is fully digested

By the end of its stay in the large intestine (12– 48 hours), most of the water content has been absorbed

Stools and gas are stored in the rectum until they are expelled through the anus

KEY POINTS

- The bowels – the large intestine – comprise the colon, the rectum and the anal canal. The only bit we consciously control is the anal canal.
- The lining of the large intestine absorbs water and salts, and repels bacteria and viruses.
- To aid absorption, the bowels constantly move the contents back and forth as well as downwards.
- Intestinal bacteria are a valuable defence against disease, even though they produce gas as well.
- How often we open our bowels varies greatly; most of us do not have a precise, 24-hour cycle.
- Many aspects of the bowels are still a mystery, even to doctors.

What affects the bowels?

Many factors in our daily lives have a direct influence on our bowels and their successful functions. These factors include our emotional state, the time of day and the amount of fibre, starch and possibly alcohol in our diet.

MORNING ROUTINE

The most important time of the day as far as the bowel is concerned is the first hour after you get up in the morning. Getting up from bed sends a wake-up message to the muscles of the colon. They begin a series of movements, known as mass peristalsis, which drives the contents of the colon towards the rectum. In some people, the drive is so powerful that the rectum fills and, within minutes of getting out of bed, they get an urge to go. In many people, however, the wake-up effect on the colon is less strong and has to be reinforced by breakfast. Eating food at any time of the day rouses the colon as well as the stomach.

EARLY MORNING CALL
For some people, the act of waking up rouses the bowel into action. Others need the reinforcement of breakfast.

23

Now comes the importance of morning routine. If the urge to go before or after breakfast is strong, well and good – it is unlikely to be ignored. However, if the feeling is less powerful so that the person is not forced to go and she (it is more often she than he) happens to be in a hurry or a flap, then the urge is liable to be ignored.

The urge is also liable to be ignored if it delays its appearance till half an hour after breakfast, or later. By then, busy people are in the thick of the day's activities or on a journey to work and often they cannot get to a loo. So they suppress the 'call to stool'. It goes away and does not come back for several hours or even for a whole day.

Obeying the call to stool is the first essential for getting a regular bowel habit and having a regular routine each morning is the best way of making sure you can obey the call. A call to stool which is regularly expected and regularly acted on is most likely to make its appearance regularly.

MORNING ROUTINE
Eating breakfast will usually stimulate the urge to defecate in many people. If ignored, it may not return for several hours or until the next meal is eaten.

THE EMOTIONS

The colon is probably more sensitive to psychological and emotional states than any other part of the body. Acute anxiety often speeds up the transit of its contents and can result in loose stools. On the other hand, any change in routine, such as travelling, can completely abolish the usual after-breakfast need to open the bowels and may lead to constipation for a day or two.

Stress and bottled-up emotions like fear, anger and resentment can have widely differing effects – in some people less frequent bowel movements and lumpier stools, in others more frequent movements and looser stools. Many people under stress develop the discomforts of the irritable bowel syndrome (see pp.56–62). They then become anxious about their insides and this causes further disturbances of gut function, especially as they may be too shy to discuss it with anyone.

There is no doubt that the stresses and strains, the haste and bustle, and the clock-watching of modern living take their toll of many people's colons. This is made harder to bear by the taboo in polite society on talking about one's bowels. It is not surprising that some people do become unhealthily obsessed with their bowels and resort to taking laxatives and other drugs. More women than men attend hospital with these problems. The links between the mind and the bowel are so important that there is a section devoted to them later in this book (see pp.63–73).

WALK TO HEALTH
Physical activity may help to prevent constipation. Keeping mobile seems to help to keep the bowel active, too.

PHYSICAL EXERCISE

Many people become constipated if they are confined to bed because of illness or injury. At the other extreme, marathon runners sometimes get diarrhoea during a race.

It is widely believed that being physically active helps to prevent constipation, but the scientific evidence is meagre. All the same, however, physical activity has many other benefits and is to be encouraged on general health grounds.

DIETARY FIBRE AND STARCH

Of all the things we eat and drink, the only ones that affect the workings of the large intestine, at least in most people, are dietary fibre, starch and, perhaps, alcohol. By dietary fibre I mean the cell walls of plants.

What dietary fibre and starch have in common is that we do not digest them completely in the small intestine, so some reaches the colon. Fibre is not digested at all, whereas starch is 90 per cent digested. However, since our diets contain about 10 times as much starch as fibre, roughly equal amounts of fibre and starch enter the first part of the colon, the caecum. They do so in the form of a thick, soup-like material, 1–1.5 litres (2–3 pints) of it a day. The colon converts this into a thick paste of spongy-solid material by absorbing most of the water and by a complex process called fermentation.

Fermentation is a chain of events whereby the large molecules (chemical substances) in dietary fibre and starch are broken down into small, simple ones by the bacteria in the colon. The bacteria do this in order to obtain energy for their own growth and multiplication, but there are two remarkable spin-offs – acids and gases. The gases are known to all of us because they are what we have to void in wind. They consist of hydrogen and carbon dioxide and, in some people, methane. They have no odour; odour comes from bacteria breaking down protein. The gases can, however, be inflammable!

You would not normally associate the colon with vinegar but, in fact, the main acid in vinegar, acetic acid, is also the main acid in the colon. Together with two others, acetic acid is responsible for the fact that the right side of the colon, where most of the fermentation takes

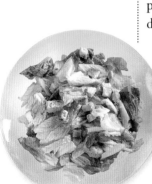

FIBRE-RICH SALAD
Although salad vegetables, such as lettuce, contain a high proportion of water, they also provide a valuable source of fibre in the diet.

place, is so acid that lots of bacteria cannot live there and others are slowed right down. In fact, this acidity may be one of the body's defences against harmful bacteria, like those that cause dysentery. One of the acids is also used as an energy source by the cells which line the colon.

Because of all this, scientists are coming round to the idea that, to stay healthy, the colon needs lots of fermentable carbohydrate going into it. This implies that our diet should contain lots of not-too-easily digestible starch or lots of fibre (except for a few people with unusually sensitive colons). One benefit is a plentiful supply of acids; the other is that stools are bulkier and softer, which makes them easier to pass.

The laxative effect of fibre has been known since antiquity but, curiously, we still do not fully understand it. Several different things probably happen. One is that fibre acts like a sponge – it is good at holding water. Another is that it tickles the nerve endings in the bowel wall, setting off electrical circuits or reflexes which make the bowel contract. A third way is that it provides a feast for the bacteria in the bowel, which then multiply furiously and add themselves to the outgoing stool. Thus, fibre is three things to the colon, all beginning with the letter S: a sponge, a stimulus and a sacrifice.

TYPES OF FIBRE

Plant cell walls consist mainly of huge molecules called polysaccharides. These are formed from lots of small sugar molecules joined end to end (Greek: poly = many, saccharides = sugars). The same is true of starch, but with starch the links between the sugars are easily split. With non-starch polysaccharides, the sugar links are hard to split; bacteria can do it, but our digestive enzymes cannot.

Some non-starch polysaccharides are like long threads or filaments. Cellulose is the prime example. Cotton is almost pure cellulose. Other non-starch polysaccharides, in fact most of them, have a branching structure which means they behave like gums or jellies. The pectin in fruit, which makes jellies set, is a familiar example.

SOURCES OF FIBRE

All foods derived from plants contain fibre, provided they have not been savagely processed. In fact, the only plant-based foods which don't contain fibre are oils, sugars and syrups. However, a lot of the fibre is removed in the milling of white flour and white rice, and in making cornflour and cornflakes.

Seeds are the best sources of fibre provided the seed-coats remain intact. So, the really fibre-rich foods are wholemeal bread and other foods made with wholemeal flour, whole-grain breakfast cereals, nuts, peas, beans and lentils.

Fruit an0d vegetables are mostly composed of water so, weight for weight, they are low in fibre. However, the British tend to eat them in fairly large amounts (especially potatoes), so they actually make an important contribution to our fibre intake.

Tables showing the fibre content of different foods are unreliable as a guide to their laxative effect. People vary hugely in how foods affect them. Foods vary hugely in their effects depending on how they have been handled and cooked, and even on how old or ripe they are. So, to get the right amount of fibre, it is best to depend on some healthy general principles: keep down your intake of oils, sugars and syrups (and animal fats) and keep up your intake of unprocessed or lightly processed plant foods. Some people's colons need more fibre than they can easily get from food, even from wholegrain cereal, and to avoid constipation they should supplement their diet with bran (see Glossary, p.84). Bran comes in many forms, some of which are very palatable. Natural, raw bran and Trifyba are probably the most effective kinds. A simple, pleasant and cheap way of taking natural bran is to mix it with porridge, muesli or another breakfast cereal. Bran also mixes well with thick soups, stewed apples, rice or yoghurt, and quite well with natural orange juice. But don't spoil a nicely presented meal by sprinkling bran all over it! Natural bran is available at health food shops and some supermarkets and chemists.

OVERDOING FIBRE

As with anything else, it is possible to take too much fibre. Some high-fibre foods upset some people, making them feel bloated and uncomfortable or giving them diarrhoea. In these cases people should use their common sense, eliminate that particular food from their diet and try a different food. If you are one of these sensitive people and suffer a bad reaction to a certain food, make sure you allow your gut time to recover fully before you include a different fibre-rich food in your diet.

Yet another way of getting into trouble with fibre is to increase your intake too quickly. If you are thinking of changing your diet, do it gradually so that your gut has time to get used to the new foods, or balance of foods, that you are introducing. If you want to take a natural bran, start with a small dose, say one flat dessertspoonful a day, and increase it gradually over two to four weeks until you achieve the desired effect. If you

Amounts of Fibre Contained in Some Foods

CATEGORY OF FOOD AND AVERAGE PORTION SIZE	FIBRE PER PORTION (G)	FIBRE PER 100 G (G)
BREAKFAST CEREALS		
Bran-based cereals (42 g)	10.5	25.0
Wheat flakes and biscuit (42 g)	5.0	12.0
Muesli-type, oat and crunchy (70 g)	5.0	7.0
Puffed rice and flaked corn cereals (28 g)	2.0	7.0
BREAD (70 G – 2 SLICES)		
Wholemeal or rye	6.0	8.5
Brown or malted wheatgrain (e.g., 'Granary')	3.5	5.0
RICE AND SPAGHETTI (56 G DRY WEIGHT)		
Brown rice	2.5	4.5
Wholemeal pasta	5.5	10.0
FRUIT AND NUTS		
Dried fruit (56 g)	9.0	17.0
Fresh fruit – 1 large piece of fruit (170 g)	4.0	2.5
Soft fruit, e.g., strawberries and apricots (113 g)	2.0	2.0
Nuts (50 g)	4.5	9.0

Amounts of Fibre Contained in Some Foods (cont'd)

CATEGORY OF FOOD AND AVERAGE PORTION SIZE	FIBRE PER PORTION (G)	FIBRE PER 100 G (G)
VEGETABLES		
Spinach (113 g)	7.0	6.0
Sweetcorn kernels (99 g)	6.0	6.0
Green leafy vegetables, broccoli and green beans (113 g)	3.0	3.0
Root vegetables, e.g., carrots, parsnips or swedes (113 g)	3.0	3.0
Salad and other watery vegetables like lettuce and cucumber (113 g)	up to 2.0	up to 2.0
Baked potato with skin (200 g)	4.0	2.0
Chips (140 g)	1.5	1.0
Boiled/mashed potato (113 g)	1.0	1.0
PULSES (113 G COOKED WEIGHT)		
Peas	13.5	12.0
Baked beans	8.2	7.3
Butter beans, kidney beans, lentils	7.0	6.0

31

find that you need more than six dessertspoonfuls a day, you should consult your doctor about alternatives.

If natural bran upsets you, try taking it in a different guise such as bran-enriched bread (for example, Hi-Bran), biscuits or cereals (several brands) or even bran tablets. If you find that your gut is intolerant of any type of bran, then you should see your doctor. Anyone who is increasing their intake of fibre should expect to pass more wind, but this unwanted side effect usually diminishes after a few weeks.

People often ask how they can check whether they are taking enough fibre. The answer is simple: just look at your stools every day for a week; if they are usually Type 4, 5 or 6 (see Bristol Stool Form Scale, p.19), you are certainly having enough and do not need to take any more. If they are always Type 3 or less, it is worth increasing your fibre intake until sometimes, at least, your stools are Type 4.

EATING ENOUGH FIBRE
There are many high-bran foods available, including bran-rich biscuits, bread, breakfast cereals and bran tablets. Be careful, however, not to overdo your intake.

KEY POINTS

- Try to establish a morning routine – this is what your bowels naturally prefer.
- Bowels are sensitive to stress and disruption of routine.
- Plenty of fibre and starch in the diet:
  - make the stools bulkier and easier to pass;
  - act as a laxative;
  - encourage the production of disease-preventing acids.
- Fibre comes from plant cell walls and is available naturally in the diet from unprocessed plant food.

What can go wrong?

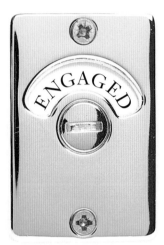

RELIEF OR FRUSTRATION?
For many people, a visit to the lavatory fails to bring the relief that it should, as they have difficulty in starting or finishing the job.

When everything goes right, opening the bowels is one of the minor pleasures of life. As with a good scratch, a discomfort is relieved; what is left is a vague, warm feeling of satisfaction. In an ideal world this brief but pleasant experience would be our lot once or twice a day – after getting up in the morning or after breakfast and, perhaps, after another meal. The act of defecation would be predictable and effortless – quickly done and quickly forgotten.

The reality is quite different. In a recent survey, a regular once or twice-a-day habit was enjoyed by less than half the men and by barely a third of the women. A unique feature of this survey was that people kept records of what actually happened after they closed the lavatory door. When all the records were analysed, several things were discovered. One discovery was that getting started was often an effort; nearly half the time people were having to hold their breath and push or strain. Finishing the job was also unsatisfactory; often the passage of the stool left a feeling that the bowel had not emptied itself properly. In fact, when some of the women volunteered to keep records for a month, it turned out that every single one experienced this feeling of rectal dissatisfaction at some time in the month, and several women were having it nearly every time they went. The natural reaction to this feeling is to keep straining in the hope that something else will come away. But it doesn't! So there must be a lot of frustrated people behind those closed doors.

Another feeling which makes people strain is a feeling of needing to go but not being able to; when they try, they can't – there's nothing there! I suspect such false alarms are a common experience but, oddly, they have not been recognised as a symptom by the medical profession. At all events, this feeling adds to the widespread impression that defecation is an act which is unpredictable and uncomfortable – at best, a nuisance and, at worst, a nightmare.

That this impression exists is very odd. No other function of the body (except, perhaps, menstruation) regularly evokes such difficulty and such distress. We breathe unconsciously (except maybe after strenuous exercise), we eat and drink automatically or with pleasure, we usually urinate without thinking about it. Why should defecation be so different?

There are several reasons, and it is important to understand them if one is to make sense of irritable bowel syndrome (IBS) and all the lesser miseries mentioned below.

COMING OUT OF THE CLOSET

Defecation is the one human function that cannot be discussed in public, let alone shown on television, although it is a good deal more natural than some of the things which are shown on television. When defecation is mentioned, it is with a snigger, a giggle, a laugh or a leer. All this makes it extremely difficult for someone who has a problem with defecation, or who just thinks they may have a problem, to mention it to anyone else. Fear of ridicule is a great conversation-stopper. So is embarrassed silence.

Another problem with talking about defecation is that, for once, the English language is totally inadequate. Let us suppose someone decides to go to their doctor and discuss what is troubling them. What do they say? Usually, it is something roundabout or very vague like 'I can't go properly'. A retired headmaster, who should have been a model of precise speech, came to me and said 'Doctor, I have great difficulty doing anything serious with my insides'. After several questions, he admitted that what he meant was that he had to strain to defecate! I suppose he may have been embarrassed to speak more

SHARE YOUR PROBLEM
If your doctor is to help you with a bowel problem, you need to explain clearly the nature of the problem.

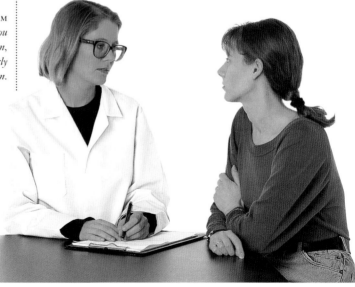

plainly but I suspect he just didn't know how to put his problem into words. Another highly educated patient, a retired lawyer, had diarrhoea. When asked to write down his complaints what he wrote was 'Uncooperative activities of alimentary canal'. People with diarrhoea usually say they have an 'upset tummy'. Again, this could mean anything.

Common Problems with the Act of Defecation

Let us suppose then that the doctor has worked out that the patient has a problem with passing stools. How then does the interview go? Rather badly in many cases, I suspect. When the patient says 'I can't go properly' they could mean at least four different things. Some common symptoms are given in the box shown on the right.

- Straining when starting to pass a stool
- Not getting an urge to go as often as expected (the technical name for this urge is the 'call to stool')
- Getting false alarms – in other words, unproductive calls to stool
- A sensation of something still inside the rectum after having passed a stool

It is important for the patient to get across to the doctor what they really mean because the first two symptoms – straining and inadequate urges – generally mean the stool is abnormally small or hard, in other words, there is constipation. The last two symptoms can be due to constipation but are more often the result of an irritable rectum. A rectum can become irritable because it is inflamed (proctitis) or because a patient has irritable bowel syndrome. So there are three possibilities. Sorting them out is important because treatment for constipation won't help proctitis and it can even make someone with IBS worse.

I wish I could say that all doctors are trained to sort out these problems, but I am afraid it would not be true. Medical textbooks are largely silent on the subject of stools and defecation, and medical students are taught

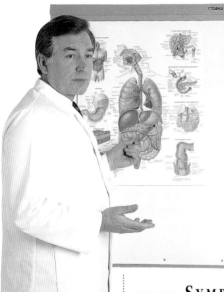

practically nothing about what is normal and what is abnormal. It is surprisingly rare for doctors, even specialists, to discuss these matters. There are some bowel symptoms which have never been given a name and others whose definition is different in different dictionaries or textbooks. This unsatisfactory situation has arisen because very little scientific work has been done in the area of defecation and stools, so this part of medicine must be considered underdeveloped.

SYMPTOMS OF DISORDER

PROBLEMS WITH DIAGNOSIS
Although medical students learn about how the bowel functions, very little is taught about stools and the process of defecation. This means that many doctors still have difficulty recognising and diagnosing abnormalities.

When the bowel is diseased or malfunctioning, the disorder usually draws attention to itself in one or more of the following ways:

- Pain in the abdomen (tummy);
- Pain in the rectum or anus (back passage);
- Bloated feelings or actual swelling of the abdomen;
- Difficult passage of stools;
- Hard stools;
- Less frequent passage of stools;
- More frequent passage of stools;
- Loose stools;
- Feelings of incomplete emptying of the rectum;
- Urgency of need to pass stools;
- Passage of blood with the stool;
- Passage of mucus (slime) from the rectum;
- Appearance of a lump in the anus.

KEY POINTS

- Easy, regular passing of stools is a pleasure denied to most of us on at least some occasions in our lives.
- Embarrassment about discussing bowel problems makes it difficult for the doctor to do something about them.
- Problems can be caused by:
  - constipation;
  - inflamed rectum;
  - irritable bowel syndrome (IBS);
  - rarer and serious diseases.

Constipation

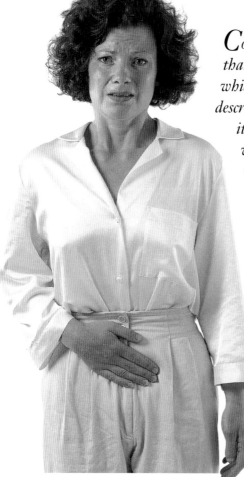

Constipation is one of those words that everyone understands but which is hard to define. It is often described as a symptom but, at best, it is a group of symptoms which vary from person to person and which have other causes besides constipation.

It is probably best defined as the state in which two things are objectively and measurably wrong: the output of stool is too low and the rate of passage of the intestine's contents is too slow. Too low and too slow. This definition is, unfortunately, no use in everyday life.

Calculating stool output and passage time with any accuracy is just too difficult. Luckily, there is a third feature of constipation that is objective but is also easy to observe – the form or appearance of the stools. In constipation the stool is lumpy – Type 1 or Type 2 on the Bristol Stool Form Scale (see p.19). But there is a

GENERAL DISCOMFORT
Constipation can often be accompanied by abdominal pain and a bloated feeling.

40

paradox. Most people who pass Type 1 or Type 2 stools do not suffer any symptoms and do not consider themselves constipated. They are, but they don't know they are. On the other hand, many people who think they are constipated are not. They have the symptoms that can go with constipation – straining, unproductive calls to stool, feelings of incomplete emptying, abdominal pain and bloating – but their symptoms are due to irritable bowel syndrome (see pp.56–62).

Apart from the form of the stools, the only reliable pointer to the state of constipation is infrequent defecation. Anyone who goes less than three times a week has slow transit. However, going more often is no guarantee that transit time is normal. It is possible to go every day, but every day be passing a stool which should have been passed three days before! There are even people who pass small, round lumps several times a day and think they have diarrhoea. What they really have is constipation and an irritable bowel.

Constipation is more common in women then in men. It is worse in pregnancy and just before a period, which are the times when the female sex hormone levels in the blood are at their highest. Severe, continuous constipation is almost unheard of in men, but affects at least one in 200 young women.

It is widely believed that constipation gets commoner as people get older. This is simply not true. It is the things that tend to go with old age which cause constipation, namely immobility and smaller food intake or the drugs which older people so often have to take.

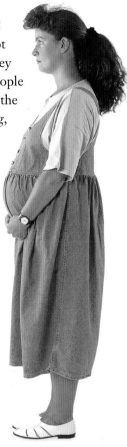

PREGNANCY PROBLEM
Virtually every pregnant woman experiences constipation at some stage. Hormonal changes make the bowel sluggish.

SMALL, LUMPY STOOLS

A small stool does not stretch the rectum enough to generate a clear signal that you need to go; the call to stool is weak. When the call is weak, many people do not bother to go to the toilet.

This is bad news because an ignored call goes away. What probably happens is that the spurned stool 'takes umbrage' and goes back up into the colon. Here it dries out and shrinks even more. Being smaller, it needs reinforcements before it is big enough to generate a signal when it descends into the rectum again. Getting reinforcements takes time, so it is often several hours, sometimes a whole day, before another call to stool is felt. Ignoring the call to stool or resisting it can definitely cause constipation. This has recently been proven in some noble volunteers!

The smaller a stool is, the more difficult it is to pass. It is as if the rectal muscles cannot get hold of it, rather like a coin which is too small for fingers to hold. When a small stool expands by reinforcement over 24 hours it can turn into a hard, dry ball. Such a ball can be hard to pass. Moreover, it can split the lining of the anal canal and lead to pain and bleeding (see p.74).

Straining – that is, holding the breath and pushing down – is often the only way to get rid of lumpy stools, but straining can be overdone. If you strain too hard or too long you can push out the soft cushions which seal the anal canal so that they protrude from the anus. This is what haemorrhoids are. Occasionally, even the lining of the rectum can be pushed out (rectal prolapse). So straining should be avoided or kept as brief as possible.

A small rectal prolapse is particularly pernicious because, as it sits in the anal canal, it can make you feel

What Goes Wrong in Constipation

Constipation is caused mainly by faeces spending too long in the colon. During this extended period of time, the body absorbs water from the faeces, making them hard, dry and difficult to propel and expel.

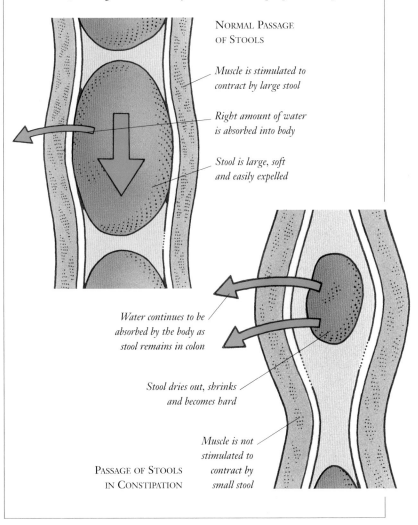

NORMAL PASSAGE
OF STOOLS

Muscle is stimulated to contract by large stool

Right amount of water is absorbed into body

Stool is large, soft and easily expelled

Water continues to be absorbed by the body as stool remains in colon

Stool dries out, shrinks and becomes hard

PASSAGE OF STOOLS
IN CONSTIPATION

Muscle is not stimulated to contract by small stool

Tips to Avoid Constipation

If you know you have a tendency to be constipated, you may find that some of the following measures help you.

- Never ignore the feeling that you need to open your bowels – a suppressed call to stool can take many hours to return.
- If possible, have a regular routine in the morning.
- Allow your bowels time to work in the morning.
- Eat breakfast. Here are some breakfast ideas: a bowl of Weetabix, Shredded Wheat, wheat flakes, bran flakes, All-Bran or branshells; a bowl of muesli with a tablespoonful of natural bran mixed into it; wholemeal bread or toast from a dense, chewy loaf (like organic stoneground or home-made bread).
- Keep up your intake of fibre, especially wheat fibre.
- If your lavatory seat is high, try putting your feet on a box or pile of books.
- If you're travelling, take some bran or packeted bulking agent (Trifyba, Isogel, Fybogel, Regulan).

as if a stool is still there. So you keep straining, which makes matters worse. This may be why some people with small stools never feel they have emptied their bowel completely.

COPING WITH THIS PROBLEM

Prevention is better than cure and there are several things you can do if you have small, lumpy stools:

1 Always obey the call to stool; in other words, if you feel the urge to go, go! Don't suppress it or delay going for more than a few minutes.

2 If possible, have a regular early morning routine so that what you do and when you do it is the same in the first hour after getting up every day.

3 Give yourself time to have a bowel movement in the morning before leaving home. If necessary, get up half an hour earlier.

4 Eat breakfast. This is normally the best way of stimulating a bowel movement successfully.

5 Let your breakfast be substantial and rich in fibre. Some examples of such a breakfast are listed in the box opposite. Any of these can be usefully supplemented with an apple or other fresh fruit (not just fruit juice) or some stewed dried fruit. Prunes are especially effective.

6 Make sure that the rest of your meals are rich in fibre (see pp.26–31).

7 A tip about coping with the difficulty in evacuation which so often results from the stool being small or hard: when sitting on the loo, try placing your feet on a platform 4 to 8 inches high so that your thighs are nearer your chest. This makes the position nearer the squatting posture which is the most natural one (as in traditional French loos).

In some people small, lumpy stools are a reaction to stress or – more accurately – a sign of emotional tension. People who have a physical reaction like this may often be dogged, determined types who are not able to show their emotions readily. It is as if, by holding on to their emotions, they can also hold on to their motions! Their gut reaction to stress is to slow down the passage of waste through the colon. If you are a person who reacts like this, then you will improve only if you manage to get rid of your tension or distress.

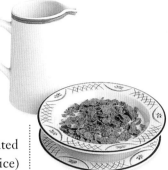

To Start the Day
Making a habit of eating breakfast, especially one that is high in fibre, can be an effective way of avoiding or alleviating constipation.

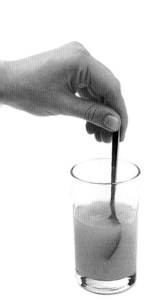

Using Laxatives

Anything that speeds up the passage of bowel contents and makes the stools softer or looser can be called a laxative. Other names for these things are aperients, purgatives and opening medicines, but these names are usually reserved for the stronger types of laxative.

The most natural laxatives are the ones that work in the same way as dietary fibre – the so-called bulking agents. They are also the safest as they hardly ever cause watery diarrhoea. There is little to choose between them except for palatability and convenience.

Several popular ones are available in handy sachets (Trifyba, Fybogel, Regulan, Normacol) or tablets (Celevac). It is reasonable for someone who thinks they are suffering from constipation to first try bran or one of the bulking agents before consulting a doctor or pharmacist.

If you try a bulking agent, remember it works slowly. Take it for at least a week before deciding whether it is working. If a small dose, say two sachets a day, does not work, try three or four a day for another week before giving up. You may feel bloated for the first few weeks but this feeling often passes.

There is a huge variety of stronger laxatives, many of which are based on traditional herbal remedies. However, don't be fooled into thinking that because a remedy is herbal in origin, and therefore 'natural', it is necessarily safe. Some have drastic effects and can make you quite ill. It is better to take a pill containing the purified active ingredient in an exactly measured, standard dose than to take pot luck with an infusion of some dried leaves or seed-pods. If you cannot see a doctor and are sure you need a strong laxative, ask the

HELPING YOURSELF
Bulking agents, which are high in fibre, offer a non-drug solution to constipation. A common type that can be bought over-the-counter comes in sachets of powder that are mixed with water to make a palatable drink.

chemist for a few senna tablets or bisacodyl tablets. Avoid anything containing phenolphthalein, including chocolate products. But if you keep needing these strong laxatives you need to have medical advice.

If you go to see a doctor about constipation, keep a record of all your bowel movements for a week or two beforehand and show it to him or her. Write down the date and time of each bowel movement and the type of each stool using the Bristol Stool Form Scale (see p.19); if a stool is part one type and part another, write down both types. Make a note of how much you have to strain, that is, hold your breath and push down. If it is longer than a minute or two, time it with your watch. Tell the doctor about any feelings of incomplete emptying and, if you are a woman, about variations in your bowel habit according to the time of the month. If you have recently taken any drugs or medicines (including laxatives) take them along with you or, at least, details of their names and doses.

KEEP A RECORD
Make a note of your bowel movements using the Bristol Stool Form Scale. This will enable you to provide the doctor with accurate information.

47

LAXATIVE RESISTANCE

In recent years it has become recognised that some women (and, rarely, men) cannot defecate because they cannot relax the muscles in the floor of the pelvis which keep the anal canal closed. In short, they cannot let go. They may also strain in an odd way so that pressures generated by straining do not go down into the pelvis. It is almost as if they are denying or rejecting this part of their anatomy. The reasons may lie deep in their unconscious mind. In any event, ordinary treatments do not help these women. Extra fibre just makes them bloated. Laxatives just cause pain or work only if taken in such big doses as to cause diarrhoea.

There is a treatment which helps such women. It is re-training their abdominal and pelvic muscles so that they cooperate instead of fighting against each other. Unfortunately, this re-training treatment is not available on the NHS, except in a few specialised centres.

However, the situation should improve as the value of this re-training treatment becomes accepted by more and more doctors and, more importantly, by funding bodies.

Another reason why some women cannot push out a stool they know to be there is that, when they strain, the rectal wall bulges forward into the vagina and the stool gets jammed in the bulge. This is called a rectocele and it can only be cured by a surgical operation.

KEY POINTS

- You are constipated if you pass lumpy or hard stools and you have no regular routine.
- To avoid constipation:
  - never ignore the call to stool;
  - establish a morning routine;
  - eat plenty of fibre.
- Laxatives: start with the bulking agents – mildest but slowest – before moving onto the stronger ones. Ask your pharmacist.
- See your doctor if you need strong laxatives regularly.
- Go to your doctor if you develop constipation for no apparent reason, especially if you are over 40. See p.77 for what might happen next.

Diarrhoea

Diarrhoea is a common disorder characterised by the passage of excessive quantities of liquid faecal matter. It has many causes, including certain foods, contaminated food or water, some drugs and emotional upset.

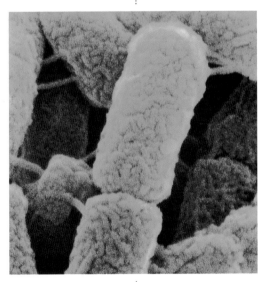

HARMFUL BACTERIA
E. coli *bacteria normally live in your intestines without causing problems. Overseas travellers are often exposed to new strains of these bacteria, which can lead to diarrhoea.*

Diarrhoea is the passing of liquid faeces, that is, mushy or watery stools, Type 6 or 7 on the Bristol Stool Form Scale (see p.19). Frequent visits to the loo do not necessarily indicate diarrhoea, unless the stools are liquid as well. Having to go frequently to pass solid stools is quite common and is a symptom of irritable bowel syndrome. It can be called pseudodiarrhoea. The distinction is very important because, in terms of cause and treatment, pseudodiarrhoea and true diarrhoea are quite different. To the sufferer who never looks into the toilet bowl they may seem exactly the same. To the doctor the appearance of the stool is all-important so, if you plan to visit a doctor about what seems like diarrhoea, make a note of what you see in the toilet bowl before you go.

How Increased Contractions Cause Diarrhoea

When muscular contractions increase in frequency and force, liquid and semi-liquid contents are forced to pass more quickly through the colon. This is often caused by food poisoning, but can also be due to stress or food intolerance.

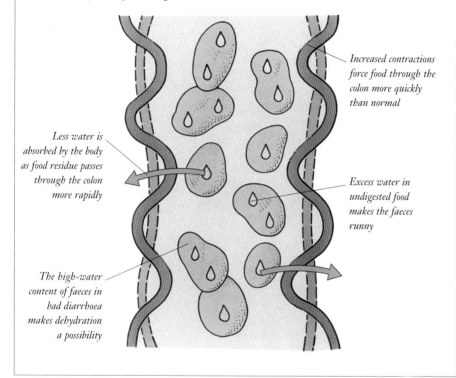

Increased contractions force food through the colon more quickly than normal

Less water is absorbed by the body as food residue passes through the colon more rapidly

Excess water in undigested food makes the faeces runny

The high-water content of faeces in bad diarrhoea makes dehydration a possibility

Liquid faeces are liquid because they have travelled fast through the colon, whose job it is to absorb water and salts, or – much less commonly – because the colon is diseased. Liquid stools are bulky and when they arrive in the rectum, you know about it at once, in no uncertain terms. The call to stool is so strong it can be painful. You have to drop everything and go to the toilet at once. Technically called urgency of defecation, this symptom causes much distress, destroying social life and self-confidence.

An even more distressing result of diarrhoea is incontinence, or soiling of the underclothes. It occurs because liquid seeps through the anus or, in the worst scenario, because the sufferer cannot get to the loo in time – the rectal muscles have been too strong for the closing mechanisms of the anus. Incontinence is more common than people suppose. It is so embarrassing and disgusting to the sufferer that most do not mention it to their doctor unless asked directly (and many doctors do not ask).

▪ COPING WITH DIARRHOEA ▪

A single watery stool which spatters the pan is no cause for concern. Several such stools are what I mean by an attack of diarrhoea.

Luckily, most attacks settle by themselves. They settle more quickly if you lie down, keep warm and avoid solid food for a few hours or a day or two. If the attack does not stop in three or four hours it is sensible to take an anti-diarrhoea tablet like loperamide (Imodium), but the most important thing is to keep up your fluid intake so that you do not become dehydrated.

Water is absorbed best if it contains a little sugar and salt. Chemist shops sell powders and effervescent tablets containing balanced amounts of sugar and salts, such as Dioralyte and Rehydrate, and these come with full instructions. In an emergency you can drink flat lemonade. If you suffer from repeated vomiting as well as diarrhoea you should get medical help urgently, and if the

REPLACING BODY FLUIDS
Diarrhoea can soon cause dehydration. Make sure that you drink plenty of water or rehydration solution to replace lost fluids.

diarrhoea persists for more than a few days, you should also see a doctor.

REPEATED DIARRHOEA

Diarrhoea which keeps coming and going is most often due to irritable bowel syndrome. This basically means that healthy intestines sometimes rush their contents through. Why? There are many reasons for intestinal hurry, but the commonest is stress or anxiety. Many people get diarrhoea before an exam, an interview or any other testing, challenging experience. It is part of the normal fight-or-flight response of a healthy body – however, in some people it occurs inappropriately often. Eating the wrong foods and eating too much food can also cause intestinal hurry. So too can alcohol in some people, especially beer in large amounts.

Intestinal hurry has many causes, and the cure must depend on the cause. Many people have a food or drink that upsets them. If you know that eating a strong curry or cabbage or drinking beer or milk leads to loose stools then, obviously, you should avoid them – unless you are happy to take the consequences! A short bout of diarrhoea is not a serious

Warning

You should seek medical advice without delay if:

- There is blood in the stool
- You are ill with fever
- The stool is black like tar

AVOIDING STRONG FOODS
If you know that hot, spicy foods such as curry give you diarrhoea, it is best to avoid eating them too frequently.

53

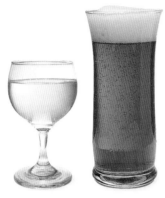

threat to your health. Persistent diarrhoea is another matter and should trigger a visit to the doctor.

If you have diarrhoea in regular bouts, and food and drink don't appear to be responsible, then ask yourself if the bouts coincide with periods of stress in your life. If so, take action to reduce the stress or get some counselling in how to handle stress better.

There are a great many complementary remedies for intestinal hurry, such as arrowroot, linseeds and herbs rich in astringent tannins. Some people believe in rice cakes and live yoghurt. None of these has been tested scientifically, but we are all different and, if something works for you and is safe, use it! Some people just need to eat less.

Should you still be prone to urgent, loose stools after doing all that you can think of, don't panic! To do so only makes things worse. To save embarrassment, plan your outings at times when you feel safest, and take a 'Can't Wait' card with you, which is available to members of the IBS Network (see p.84).

CUT DOWN ON ALCOHOL
The sugars in alcohol, especially beer, can cause diarrhoea in some people. Reduce your intake if you suffer from repeated bouts of diarrhoea.

MARSHMALLOW PLANT

DRIED TORMENTIL ROOT

NATURAL REMEDIES
The roots of the tormentil and marshmallow plants are often used in professionally made herbal medicine for treating diarrhoea.

KEY POINTS

- Diarrhoea means passing liquid faeces; it does not mean having to go to the toilet frequently.
- Most attacks settle by themselves.
- For diarrhoea which keeps coming and going, there are many possible causes, both psychological and physical. Treat it by whatever means works for you.
- Always consult a doctor if your diarrhoea is persistent (see p.77 for what is likely to happen next).

Irritable bowel syndrome (IBS)

*T*his is the name given by doctors to the
situation in which the intestine keeps
misbehaving or malfunctioning and there is no
apparent disease of the intestines to explain it.

HOW DOES IT HAPPEN?

Short, self-limiting spells of intestinal malfunction are so
common that they are part of normal life (see table, p.60).
In some people, however, the intestine continues to
malfunction long after the original cause has gone away.
If such people go to a doctor they are likely to be told
that they have IBS.

TALK TO YOUR DOCTOR
*Be as specific as you can when
describing your symptoms; this
will help the doctor to give an
accurate diagnosis.*

What has happened is that their
intestine has become sensitised, which
means made more sensitive. It has
been sensitised by the original
upset or by their psychological
reaction to the upset. The
intestine, including the rectum,
is now more easily roused
into activity than it should
be. Its activity may be
excessive, that is to say, its
muscles contract more

strongly than they should. However, the main problem is that signals from the intestine travel up the nervous system into the brain and so to the conscious mind more often than they should. These signals are registered as unpleasant feelings like pain, bloatedness, the urge to pass wind or the urge to pass stool.

Unfortunately, a vicious circle often sets in. Focusing attention on part of the body makes it easier for signals from that part to reach the conscious mind. If you have a slight itch on your back and you focus your mind on it, it becomes a stronger itch. If you have a twinge somewhere and focus on it, it can turn into a pain. All sensations from the body can be amplified by attending to them and, on the other hand, they can be damped down or even abolished by fixing your attention on something else. The sensations coming from the bowel are harder to ignore than itches and twinges because they have an alarming or embarrassing quality. Unfortunately, being alarmed or embarrassed is all too often the first step in focusing the mind on the bowel and so, quite unintentionally, making it more sensitive. A later section of this booklet on the mind and the bowel (pp.63–73) elaborates on this important point.

COULD IT BE SERIOUS?

Many people who go to a doctor with IBS are afraid there is something seriously wrong like cancer, colitis, ulcers or AIDS. Such fear is misplaced. The symptoms of IBS have lots of features which show that the problem is a functional one and is not due to serious disease.

1 The symptoms usually come and go over hours or days. For example, bloating or swelling of the abdomen gets worse as the day goes on but disappears overnight.

In serious disease the symptoms are persistent. There are a few exceptions like the pain of gallbladder stones, but such stones are not life threatening anyway.

2 The symptoms of IBS vary in kind from time to time. For example, the pain is often felt in different places, or the stools may vary in appearance from day to day. In serious disease the symptoms tend to be stereotyped.

3 The pains of IBS have features which show that they come from the intestine. For example, they may ease off when the bowels are opened. Commonly, someone with IBS has a change in bowel habit at a time when the pains are occurring; typically the stools become softer or more frequent. Paradoxically, this change is sometimes welcomed – that is, in people with a tendency to constipation. Of course there are serious diseases which can cause intestinal pain and a change of habit, but they are rare compared with IBS and are usually obvious in some other way, for example, by bleeding or vomiting.

4 In IBS there are often symptoms of an irritable rectum; these are unproductive calls to stool ('want to but can't'), urgent calls to stool and feelings after you have defecated that there is still something inside the rectum. (With the latter feeling there is a natural tendency to keep straining but this should be resisted as it can make matters worse.) Serious disease rarely causes these symptoms and, when it does, it will also cause anal bleeding.

5 You may see slime (mucus) on the stool or even have occasions when you pass nothing but slime. This is nothing to worry about unless it is copious or there

Getting Enough Rest
Many of the symptoms of IBS disappear after a good night's sleep.

is blood too. It is simply the reaction of an irritated rectum.

6 Some people with IBS notice they have to pass urine more often. This is a sign that the bladder has become more sensitive, like the intestine. In women, the womb and surrounding areas may get more sensitive too so that sexual intercourse is painful.

7 In some people with IBS, the gullet and stomach get more sensitive so that they feel excessively full after normal-sized meals or get heartburn after consuming foods or drink that never used to upset them. Others get excessively hungry and tend to binge.

8 A lot of people feel tired and listless during attacks of IBS. In fact they feel generally out of sorts, perhaps getting headaches and backaches too.

So you can see that people with IBS have a lot to complain about. When it comes to seeing a doctor this multiplicity of complaints has a good side and a bad side.

The good side is that the sheer number and variety of symptoms help the doctor deduce that the problem is a functional one and not a serious disease. The downside is that some doctors find patients with functional complaints like IBS hard to handle. In attempting to reassure the patient they may let drop an unhelpful remark like 'there is nothing wrong with you'. This is incorrect.

There is something wrong but it is a misbehaviour of the intestines, not a disease in the conventional sense. IBS is a subtle and varied condition which even specialists do not fully understand. But this does not mean that nothing can be done about it.

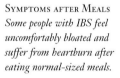

SYMPTOMS AFTER MEALS
Some people with IBS feel uncomfortably bloated and suffer from heartburn after eating normal-sized meals.

Common Causes of Short-Lived Constipation and/or Diarrhoea

The following are causes of constipation and diarrhoea of short duration. Always consult a doctor if the attack is prolonged.

CAUSE	CONSTIPATION	DIARRHOEA
MEN AND WOMEN		
Disturbed morning routine	✓	
Worrying situation	✓	✓
Change in diet	✓	✓
Alcohol, especially beer		✓
Food intolerance		✓
Travellers' diarrhoea		✓
Slimming regimes	✓	
Virus infections, gastroenteritis		✓
Antibiotic treatment		✓
Other drugs	✓	✓
WOMEN ONLY		
Before periods	✓	
During periods		✓
Pregnancy	✓	

WHAT CAN BE DONE FOR IBS?

As with all diseases and disorders of the human body and mind, treatment varies according to the severity and circumstances of the case. In many people with IBS, especially those who have recently developed it, all that is needed is to be told by the doctor exactly what is going wrong and why. This breaks the vicious cycle of gut reaction-emotional reaction, and the intestine calms down.

Some people need to change their diet. If particular foods or drinks have triggered attacks or worsened the symptoms, they should be avoided or limited till the attack is over. If there is a tendency to constipation it often helps to eat more fibre-rich foods (see pp.30–31), unless these cause bloating. Some people need to lay off coffee because it stimulates the nervous system, including the bit which controls the intestine. People who have diarrhoea without alternating constipation may be reacting to an everyday item of their diet, like wheat or dairy products. This is quite complicated to sort out, and anyone who thinks they may have this problem should see a registered dietician.

STIMULATING DRINKS
Too much coffee, tea or caffeine-containing cola drinks can make IBS symptoms worse.

Drugs can be useful in the short term but are not a permanent solution. The most commonly prescribed are bulking agents such as ispaghula, sterculia and methylcellulose, and drugs which help the bowel muscles to relax such as mebeverine, anti-muscarinics and peppermint oil preparations.

Often people with IBS benefit from alterations in lifestyle which help them to relax and cope better with the stresses of life. Regular physical exercise helps a lot of people, as do the techniques of yoga, t'ai chi and meditation. With some people, the most important thing to do is to escape from a personal relationship that is keeping them tense, angry or depressed. Other people simply need to take more time for relaxation and personal development. Each person has his or her own needs but may find it hard to look at him- or herself objectively and identify the problem area. A wise counsellor is often needed. More and more general practices now employ trained counsellors. If you want a peaceful bowel, you need a peaceful mind!

LEARN TO RELAX
Most doctors believe that stress is a contributory factor to IBS. Techniques such as yoga will relax the body and calm down the mind.

KEY POINTS

- Irritable bowel syndrome (IBS) occurs when the intestines continue to misbehave without there being any underlying disease.
- The mental attitude of the sufferer has a great influence on the severity and duration of IBS.
- Treatment can involve changes to lifestyle and diet; drugs can help in the short term.
- Any single symptom of IBS can be caused by a serious disease so, if in doubt, check with your doctor.

Mind and bowel

There is a network of interactions between the mind and the bowel, and there are many ways in which they affect each other. Some are obvious, some are subtle. Let us look at them in turn, starting with the neglected but important matter of how the bowel affects the mind.

ATTITUDES TO THE BOWELS

All the internal organs of the body are mysterious to ordinary, non-medical people but, nevertheless, they have feelings about them. Take the heart and the brain. Everyone, quite rightly, thinks that the heart and brain are marvellous inventions of nature; our feelings about these organs are positive, even warm. Again, take the womb. Women treasure the womb as the place where human life begins. Towards other organs, such as the liver and kidneys, we have no special emotions, except perhaps gratitude that

OVERACTIVE BOWELS
A stressful business meeting can cause the bowel to over-react, sometimes necessitating a hasty exit.

they quietly get on with their job. The bladder can be a source of discomfort but one that is quickly relieved and forgotten. Only the gut and the intestines evoke consistently negative emotions. Intestines are forever drawing attention to themselves in ways that embarrass or harass us. They are liable to gurgle loudly in meetings or concerts. At times they also insist on discharging a smelly gas – usually when we are in company. They demand attention unpredictably and in inconvenient places. Who has not been forced to creep shamefacedly out of a social or professional occasion because of an irresistible need to go to the toilet?

And all this is when the bowel is healthy and working normally. How much worse these things are when the bowel is diseased or malfunctioning! And everyone knows that the bowel is a place where serious diseases happen. Thanks to ex-presidents of the USA, Reagan and Bush, everyone has heard about bowel cancer and, though both men seem to have been cured, cancer is cancer and most people have heard of someone who has died of bowel cancer. Indeed, 16,000 people die of it every year in the UK. So the seeds of fear are sown and, in many people's minds, this fear grows hugely every time their bowels misbehave or they see a streak of blood on the toilet paper.

Nowhere are these negative feelings of embarrassment, shame and fear more apparent than in people's attitudes to stools and defecation. These things are unmentionable except in emotive language. To call someone 'a shit' means that you find them deeply unpleasant. One of the worst humiliations is to be exposed to someone else's faeces. The most degrading infirmity of the human body is being unable to control your own discharge of faeces.

From infancy, we are taught to fear faeces and to be ashamed of them. They are the big no-no of modern Western civilisation.

It is a truism that fear breeds hostility, and it is another truism that fear feeds on ignorance. Thanks to the nineteenth-century invention of the water closet, most people are ignorant of what human faeces look like. Some do not even know what their own stools are like. This is odd because we all know what horse manure, cow dung, sheep droppings, dog faeces and bird droppings look like. People feel little or no discomfort looking at excreta from other species but are disgusted, shocked or angered by any mention of human excreta, let alone the actual sight of them.

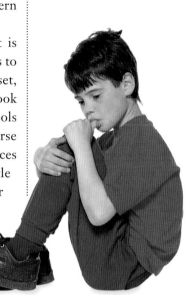

Ignorance about the act of defecation is equally profound. This normal, natural function is, simply, never discussed. Novels and biographies describe every human activity in intimate detail except for one. In books, it would appear that no one ever defecates.

FEELING ASHAMED
Negative feelings about faeces are taught in childhood and may last a lifetime.

The English language – so rich in every other way – is totally deficient here. The very word defecation is absent in Roget's Thesaurus of English Words and Phrases. The only words most people know are the crude slang words 'crap' and 'shit'. In the English-speaking world there is a conspiracy of denial.

To summarise, in our culture people's attitudes to the intestines and their products are expressed as disgust, embarrassment, shame, fear and denial. This is a potent cocktail of negative feelings to have deep in the unconscious mind. It must colour the way we react to any problems with our bowels.

HOW MIND AFFECTS BOWEL

All human beings experience strong emotions. Strong emotions can affect every function of the body. A severe shock can make a person faint; it can make their heart bump or race. Anger makes people turn red and see red. It can also turn them white and make them shake uncontrollably. Anxiety makes people feel hot while fear makes them break into a cold sweat. Knees buckle, heads spin, eyes gush fluid, mouths go dry, throats go tight, voices go hoarse – all these things happen as a result of emotion.

The effects of emotion on the body are mostly on organs that are outside our conscious control. Our intestines most certainly belong in this category. Experiments done on volunteers using telescopes, balloons and pressure-recording apparatus have proved that fear can paralyse the lower bowel and anger can work it up into a frenzy of activity. Everyday experience bears this out. The student waiting to go into an exam, the applicant before an interview, the sportsman before a match, the soldier before a battle – all are likely to have a violent urge to void a loose stool. Anxiety, which here is the anticipation of stress rather than the stress itself, has dramatically altered the function of the intestine. Another example of this same phenomenon is the acute pain in the abdomen which a child gets when it is time to go to

A STRESSFUL SITUATION
Nervous tension can affect the bowels. Many people suffer from diarrhoea when faced with a stressful situation, like a difficult deadline at work.

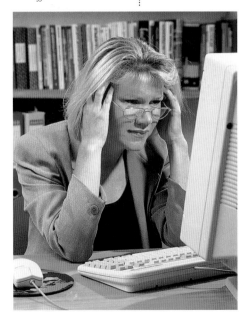

school or which a student gets when exams are looming. A person I know would get severe stomach-ache whenever her sister came to stay – a sister who irritated her and made her tense. Her stomach pains came from an intestine that had become irritable and tense.

What happens in all these examples is that emotional reactions are internalised. Elemental feelings are swallowed and are expressed inwardly rather than outwardly. Instead of fists being clenched or faces going red, the intestine clenches itself and the rectum goes red. Instead of insults or missiles being hurled, the contents of the intestine are hurled. The same things can happen in the stomach; some people react to an unpleasant or frightening scene by vomiting. A girl once saved herself from rape by vomiting on her attacker. An attack of diarrhoea might have done the trick too. This may all sound very primitive but, under our civilised veneer, we are all primitive. Our animal heritage will not be denied. We cannot help having gut reactions.

STRESS AT SCHOOL
For some children, school stresses such as examinations can cause acute stress, leading to stomach or bowel problems.

BOWELS AND LIFE'S STRESSES

Civilisation saves us from the cruder stresses of animal life or of primitive man – at least in times of peace. However, civilised life creates new stresses which are more subtle and, perhaps, more difficult to cope with. For one thing, society demands that we hide our feelings, except at funerals and football matches. We say that we are controlling ourselves, but all we are doing is hiding our feelings. Feelings cannot be wished away and, if we hide them, they will still affect us in some way. Having to control our reactions is stressful, yet failure to do so incurs disapproval or disgrace. Each person is trapped within their own personality and their own situation in life. Each has to learn coping tactics, but few of us are taught them. Talking to other people about one's feelings is often the best tactic, but some cannot do this. They may have nobody at all to talk to, or nobody they can trust to listen sympathetically. Many people, especially men, and especially northern Europeans, cannot talk about their feelings because they have learnt to deny their existence. They have buried their feelings so deep they have lost touch with them.

Not expressing feelings freely makes it more likely that the internal organs of the body will show the effects of stress – the 'slings and arrows of outrageous fortune' as Shakespeare called them. The only question is whether the slings and arrows will cause external bruises and sprains or internal ones.

A VICIOUS CIRCLE

Let us look now at what can happen when, for one reason or another, someone's intestinal function is disturbed. There are many reasons why this could happen besides a stressful event, as listed previously (see p.60). Remember the profound negative reaction that bowels and faeces induce in most of us and it is easy to see how, in some people, the fear, disgust or anxiety induced by their symptoms will affect the workings of their intestine and induce more symptoms. The continuation of the symptoms reinforces the negative emotions, especially the fear that there is something seriously wrong, and the continuing negative emotions reinforce the symptoms. And so it goes on, especially if the sufferer has a friend or relative who had cancer of the bowel. A vicious circle like this, and they are common enough in all branches of medicine, can be easily broken if the sufferer is quickly seen by a doctor or other trusted adviser who can explain the origin and meaning of the symptoms and reassure them that what they have had is a common, everyday occurrence which gets better by itself, at least if it is not worried about.

Unfortunately, this often does not happen for several reasons. One obvious one is that the sufferer from a bowel complaint is too shy or too busy to mention it to anyone. Another is failure of communication – the sufferer fails to explain the embarrassing or confusing symptoms accurately to the doctor, or the doctor misses the point or is brusque and unsympathetic, and the opportunity for reassurance is lost. This is particularly bad news because the sufferer who knows his sufferings have been misunderstood has an extra source of grievance or anxiety or guilt – 'What on earth do I do now? Why didn't he listen to me? Was it my fault? Dare I ask to see the doctor again?'. This extra layer of emotions perpetuates and strengthens the vicious cycle.

There are more subtle reasons why symptoms can persist. In a strange way they can actually make the sufferer feel better! Physical pain is easier to bear than psychic pain. If the pain started as a response

GOOD COMMUNICATION
Don't let embarrassment stand in the way – make sure that you explain your symptoms clearly and carefully to your doctor.

to life stresses it may be a substitute for anger or hatred and be easier to bear than the original raw emotion. If the cause of the anger or hatred has not been faced up to or removed, then the sufferer is unconsciously choosing to have pain rather than to feel the raw emotion.

In civilised life there are many intractable conflicts – between the older and younger generations, between employees and managers, between more time with the family and more overtime pay, and so on. Many conflicts are between opposing loyalties. Conflicts create tension, and long-standing tension can turn into chronic anxiety or depression. But in Britain, it is socially less acceptable to complain of anxiety or depression or other forms of mental pain than it is to complain of physical pain and other bodily symptoms. People with physical problems are perceived as victims of forces outside themselves and deserving of sympathy, whereas people with mental complaints are perceived as weak and just needing to pull themselves together. No wonder abdominal pain is so common. At any one time it affects one in five women and one in 10 men, and surveys show that people who admit to being troubled by pain from the intestines are mostly people who are having a hard life or a hard time coping with life.

EFFECTS OF MENTAL DISTRESS

The body's computer systems for receiving signals from the intestines, analysing them and telling the intestine what to do are immensely complex and far from fully understood. The brain, with which we register all sensations including those from the intestine, is in the frustrating position of not being able to control events in the gut, at least not directly or consciously. It has to operate through another nervous system which is wrapped round the intestine and is called the enteric nervous system or ENS. The ENS needs no help from above in controlling the intestine; in fact it functions most smoothly if left to its own devices.

There would probably be no need for this book if the mind had no influence on the intestines and vice versa! Unfortunately, mental states do affect the intestine, and they probably do so by affecting the settings of controls in the enteric nervous system.

Signals or messages coming down from the brain make the ENS more sensitive, reacting to weak stimuli as if they were strong ones. Current research suggests that the nerve endings or receptors in the intestinal wall are 'up-regulated' (the current jargon for placed on red

Nervous Control of the Digestive System

The digestive system has its own nervous system, called the enteric nervous system, which is made up of over 5 million nerve cells. Messages from our brains can occasionally cause the system to misbehave and generate bowel symptoms.

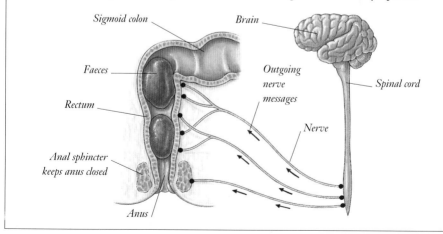

alert), but there may also be changes in the junction boxes. These appear to allow weaker than normal signals through, and the signals may even be amplified so that they get all the way up the spinal cord and so back to the brain.

There are similar junction boxes in the spinal cord where incoming signals from the intestine can get amplified when the wrong messages, or too many messages, are coming down from the brain.

The neurochemical mechanisms are not fully worked out. We do know, however, that after a time the setting of a junction box in the nervous system can become fixed so that, long after the original intestinal upset or mental problem has disappeared, the mechanisms still exist for producing abnormal sensations from the intestine. It is as if a pain or other symptom becomes imprinted on the nervous system. In this way the pain becomes chronic and intractable.

WHAT CAN BE DONE?

People can avoid vicious cycles and intractable symptoms by keeping calm and not jumping to pessimistic conclusions every time they have a pain in their tummy, a hard stool or a series of loose stools. Remember that these things are happening all the time to all kinds of people, they usually have no sinister significance and they usually go away on their own. Look at the list of common causes of short-lived intestinal malfunction (see p.60) and ask yourself if one of them seems to apply. If so, expect things to get better. If they don't or, for any other reason, you decide to see your doctor, make sure he or she really understands what you are saying is wrong with you. Make sure, too, that you understand what he or she says when explaining the nature of your problem. Don't be shy about your symptoms, and don't be afraid to ask questions. If you can't talk to your doctor, talk to some other person who you feel you can trust.

Above all, admit that you had a shock, for example, or that you are worried or are finding things hard to cope with. A trouble shared is a trouble halved.

KEY POINTS

- Thinking about our bowels encourages all the negative feelings – embarrassment, shame and fear. These lead to denial and ignorance.
- Strong emotional reactions, especially when repressed, can play havoc with the bowels.
- Beware the vicious circle: negative attitudes increase the nervous sensitivity of the bowels, magnify the feeling of intestinal discomfort and make us even more negative.
- A positive approach is therapeutic in itself. But if you have to see the doctor, tell him or her clearly and in plain English what is wrong.

Bleeding from the anus

Bleeding from the anus after passing a stool is very common. When 1,620 English people were asked about it in a survey, 10 per cent said they had noticed it in recent months. However, this is a low estimate.

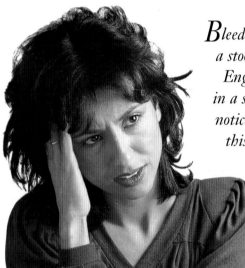

DON'T BE ALARMED
The sight of blood in the lavatory pan may cause alarm, but it is usually due to something harmless.

When people with irritable bowel syndrome, who are more observant of their stools than the rest of us but have no particular reason to bleed from the anus, were asked the same question no less than 35 per cent had seen blood.

Where does it come from? In most people the blood comes from the anal canal and there are two common causes. If there is pain in the back passage during or just after the stool is passed, then the blood probably comes from a small split or tear in the lining of the anal canal. This tends to happen when the stool is unusually broad or hard. If there is no pain then the blood most likely comes from a haemorrhoid (or pile).

A haemorrhoid is an anal cushion which has been pushed down the anal canal. It is a soft, fragile lump

74

Types of Haemorrhoid

Haemorrhoids (right) may be internal or external; normal veins are shown on the left. Internal haemorrhoids develop in the anal canal. External haemorrhoids develop on the outer edge of the anus, and may be felt when passing stools.

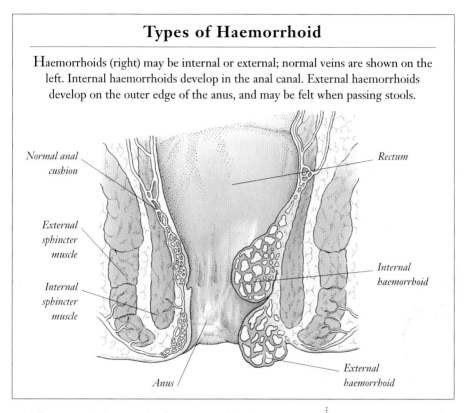

Normal anal cushion

Rectum

External sphincter muscle

Internal haemorrhoid

Internal sphincter muscle

Anus

External haemorrhoid

which is easily damaged when a stool passes over it. Often the owner of the haemorrhoid does not know it is there, but some people can feel a lump just inside or outside the anus. Although this may be uncomfortable, it should not be painful. It may ooze a slimy material – mucus. This is a nuisance because it can soil the underwear and may also lead to itching around the anus.

The bleeding from an internal haemorrhoid can appear to be quite alarming, but it is never serious. It may splash or drip into the lavatory pan or just be seen as a streak on the stool or the toilet paper.

Haemorrhoids are caused by straining to pass a stool, so are commonest in people who are constipated or who keep straining because the rectum is irritable, sending false signals that there is a stool inside.

Small haemorrhoids often go away when the constipation is cured or when straining stops. Bigger ones need treatment by a surgeon. Usually a simple injection or rubber band does the trick, but occasionally the haemorrhoid has to be cut away under general anaesthetic.

WHEN IS BLEEDING SERIOUS?

In a small minority of people bleeding is caused by a disease of the bowel higher up than the anus itself. The most serious cause is cancer of the rectum or of the lower colon, but it can also come from innocent tumours (called polyps), inflammation of the rectum (proctitis) or inflammation of the colon just above the rectum (distal colitis). All of these conditions can be cured, and cure is more likely if treatment is begun sooner rather than later.

Bleeding from these causes is often less obvious than bleeding from the anus itself and may be seen only if you inspect the stool closely. However, it is important for an ordinary person to know whether bleeding has a serious cause, so the only safe policy is to see your doctor as soon as possible. There is one exception to this rule. If the bleeding is a rare, one-off event and happens only when you have had a painful time passing an unusually broad or hard stool, then it can be safely put down to a tear of the anal lining. It is a sensible precaution for people over 50 to look at their stools occasionally, say once a month, to see if they are streaked with blood. But don't be fooled by a piece of undigested tomato skin which looks like blood!

— WHAT WILL THE DOCTOR DO? —

Some people put off going to see a doctor with a bowel complaint for fear of what may be done to them. Actually it will not be as bad as they think. It may be undignified, but it should not be painful. The doctor's examination will include feeling the tummy or abdomen with you lying on your back, not prodding it but gently probing it with the fingers, at first lightly then quite deeply, probing each part of the tummy in turn, searching for any lumps or tender places. The doctor will ask you to turn on to your left side with your knees drawn up towards your chest for the examination of the back passage. First the doctor inspects the outside of the anus, then he or she feels the inside of it. To do this the doctor lubricates his or her gloved right forefinger with jelly and gently slides it into the anal canal. At this point you can make the examination more comfortable for yourself and easier for the doctor by relaxing the muscles round the back passage. It helps if you breathe slowly and deeply with your mouth open. Having felt all round the anal canal the doctor withdraws the finger and inspects it for signs of blood. If there are faeces on the glove the doctor may make a smear on a piece of special soft paper and add a drop or two of chemical to test for invisible traces of blood (which react to give a blue colour).

If you have been bleeding, the doctor's next examination will probably be proctoscopy. This is a visual inspection of the anal canal (and lower rectum) and should really be called anoscopy. It is done with a

INVESTIGATING SYMPTOMS
As a first step in the investigation of your symptoms, your doctor will gently examine your abdomen.

four-inch long steel tube as thick as a man's finger. If you relax your anus again the tube will slide in just as easily as the finger because it is well lubricated and its business end is rounded off by a removable plug called an obturator. When the plug is pulled out a bright light shows the doctor if there are any haemorrhoids or other problems in the anal canal. These become obvious as he slowly pulls the instrument out of you. The tube may feel cold and strange but, I repeat, it should not hurt. If it does, say so at once and the doctor will stop. If further examinations are necessary, they can be done with an anaesthetic.

The next routine examination for bowel complaints, a sigmoidoscopy, is done by some GPs but not many. It is very likely to be done by the hospital specialist if you are sent to one. It is the same in principle as a proctoscopy, but the tube is longer. Most often it is 10 inches long (25 cm) so the doctor can see the whole of the rectum. Sometimes he can see further, into the sigmoid colon (hence sigmoidoscopy), but usually this is not possible because there is a sharp bend where the rectum joins the sigmoid. Sigmoidoscopy is a quick procedure (two or three minutes) but is very valuable to the doctor. During it he or she has to pump some air into the bowel. Many feel a sensation of needing to pass wind when this is being done. If it is more uncomfortable than that it suggests you have an irritable bowel. This could be the best clue to your diagnosis so, if it happens, do mention it to the doctor.

While doing a sigmoidoscopy the doctor may decide to take a snippet of tissue from the wall of the rectum – a rectal biopsy – for examination under the microscope. This is done with long forceps which are passed down the tube. Although most people do not feel it, those with a sensitive rectum may feel a tweak.

Investigating the Colon

Many abnormalities of the rectum and sigmoid colon can be seen by your doctor through a sigmoidoscope. This is a routine procedure that may cause slight discomfort, but it is unlikely to be painful.

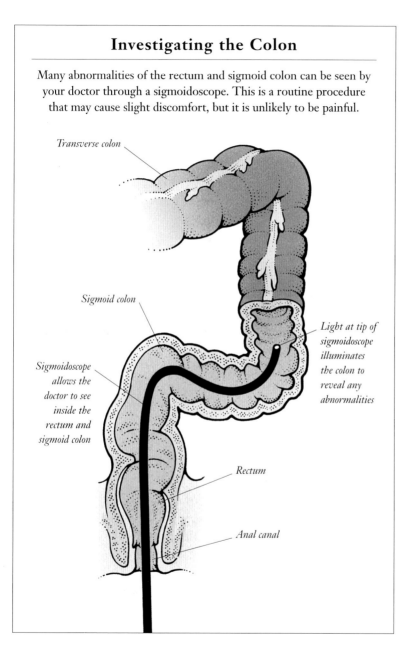

Transverse colon

Sigmoid colon

Light at tip of sigmoidoscope illuminates the colon to reveal any abnormalities

Sigmoidoscope allows the doctor to see inside the rectum and sigmoid colon

Rectum

Anal canal

79

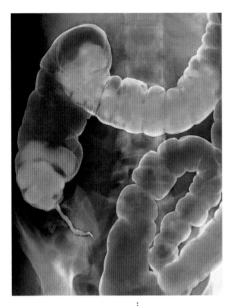

BARIUM-ENHANCED X-RAY
The use of an X-ray image of the large intestine, enhanced by a barium enema, is a common test for bowel problems. It allows the doctor to examine the walls of the colon and to look for possible polyps or tumours.

In Britain all these procedures are done without obtaining formal, written consent, but consent is usually requested before the more lengthy and specialised examination of fibreoptic endoscopy. These are done by hospital specialists using much longer flexible instruments which are called flexible sigmoidoscopes and colonoscopes. These enable the doctor to inspect the last 30 per cent and 100 per cent of the colon respectively. If you need such an examination you will be given full instructions in advance of your appointment. These will probably include taking a laxative to clean out the colon beforehand. For the examination you will be given a sedative injection to take away any discomfort.

Another common test is an X-ray with a barium enema. This also involves a hospital visit and a laxative clear-out beforehand. You will be asked to lie on your side on the X-ray table and a lubricated tube will be slid into your back passage. A liquid suspension of barium sulphate, which shows up on the X-rays, will be poured down the tube. Some air will be passed in and you will be asked to change position several times so that the barium runs all the way around your colon. X-rays will be taken and then the air and some barium will be drained out. You will then be sent to the toilet to expel the remaining barium.

Finally, remember that it is better to seek advice sooner rather than later if your bowels are causing you concern. Don't be embarrassed – it certainly won't be the first time the doctor has faced a patient with these problems.

KEY POINTS

- Bleeding from the anus is common but only rarely indicates a serious problem. Tears in the anal canal or haemorrhoids are the usual explanation.
- Be on the safe side. Unless the bleeding is a one-off event, see your doctor about it as soon as you can.
- Check regularly for blood in the stool.
- Your doctor will examine you both inside and out. The internal examination should be painless, even if an instrument (proctoscope) is used to help the doctor see better.
- Hospital specialists may examine you with longer instruments (sigmoidoscopes, colonoscopes). These should be painless procedures.
- Sometimes a barium enema X-ray is needed.

Travellers' problems

A change in bowel function is almost inevitable with travel, especially modern high-speed travel. The best-known disturbance is diarrhoea but I suspect constipation is even commoner.

CONSTIPATION

There has never been a proper investigation to settle it, but many people have told me they don't 'go' for several days whenever they are away from home. There are several reasons why this may happen. First, being away involves loss of the normal morning routine. Second, there are turn-offs to obeying the call to stool: loos are unfamiliar and hard to find or plain distasteful, and it is often quite a public business to get to the loo. This is all very intimidating to shy people. Thirdly, during long-distance travel with crossing of time zones, there is disruption of people's internal or biological clock and so of their bodily rhythms. Finally, there is a change of diet, which, for many people, means a fall in their intake of dietary fibre.

Some of this is inevitable. But there are some things you can do to prevent constipation when you are travelling. One is to choose an aisle seat on the plane or train so that you can easily and unobtrusively slip along to the loo. Another is to avoid sitting still for long periods; if you are driving, break the journey every hour or so. A third is to take along packets of high-fibre foods like rye biscuits and breakfast cereals. More

compactly, you can take sachets of Trifyba or another bulk laxative (see pp.46–47). Start to take them a day or two before you leave home. Finally, when you get a call to stool, make sure you obey it as soon as possible.

DIARRHOEA

In visitors to the middle and far east and the tropics, diarrhoea is so common it is almost regarded as inevitable and has been given many names like Delhi Belly, Nile Trots and Montezuma's Revenge. Luckily most cases are short-lived and can be coped with by avoiding solid food and lying down for a few hours and/or taking a tablet of loperamide or some kaolin mixture. If it looks like something more serious then do not delay in getting medical aid, and keep yourself hydrated.

What causes travellers' diarrhoea? Most cases are a mild attack of gastroenteritis caused by a virus or a bacterium like *E. coli* which the body can cope with on its own. Worse illnesses are likely to be due to Salmonella or Shigella infection or, perhaps a Campylobacter. They are picked up from food or drink contaminated by a foodhandler who has not washed his or her hands or by a water supply contaminated by sewage. The time-honoured way to avoid them is to drink only boiled, bottled or sterilised water and to avoid ice, ice-cream and raw fruit and salads. For further information see p.52.

Worms

In third world countries there are many kinds of worm which infest a high proportion of the population. Some cause a lot of debility and anaemia (hookworms). These worms require special tests for their detection, but fortunately they are easily cured.

THREADWORMS

In all parts of the world, children sometimes acquire worms in the intestine, probably from poor hygiene. These are called threadworms in Britain because they are seen on the surface of the stool (faeces) as small, white threads which may be seen to wriggle. (In the U.S. they are known as pinworms.) They are harmless, but in some people the female worm causes an annoying itch by escaping out of the anus to lay its eggs, especially at night. One way to prove threadworms are present is to put a piece of sticky transparent tape on the anus and put it under a microscope to see the eggs.

Threadworms are easily got rid of by a tablet containing a drug called mebendazole. It is obtainable from any doctor on prescription or over the counter from a chemist as Ovex or Pripsen Mebendazole. A single tablet is enough to kill all the worms in the intestine. It is sensible for other members of the household to take a tablet too because some people who harbour worms do so without knowing it.

Reinfection with threadworms occurs when people scratch their bottoms and then put a contaminated finger in the mouth or touch food with unwashed hands. If someone has had threadworms treated everyone in the household should wash their hands thoroughly for the next few weeks after going to the loo and, to be really safe, scrub their fingernails. Another way of preventing reinfection is to have a bath or a bidet wash immediately on rising in the morning. This gets rid of any eggs laid around the anus in the night.

Threadworms, like many other infections, can also be acquired by sexual practices involving contact with the anus.

Glossary

Anus: the lower opening of the alimentary canal or gut.

Barium enema: an X-ray procedure in which a thick, white liquid (a suspension of barium sulphate) is introduced into the colon via a tube in the anus. It is used to look for signs of colitis, polyps, etc.

Bran: the outer coats of a cereal grain, usually wheat (after the husk has been removed by winnowing). Bran is an exceptionally rich source of dietary fibre.

Colectomy: surgical removal of the colon.

Colitis: inflammation of the colon; often used as an abbreviation for ulcerative colitis.

Colonoscopy: examination of the colon by a flexible telescope (or fibreoptic endoscope) called a colonoscope, which is introduced via the anus.

Colostomy: surgical procedure in which an opening is constructed between the colon and the skin of the abdomen.

Constipation: difficulty in passing stools and/or having lumpy stools.

Crohn's disease: inflammation of part of the alimentary canal, usually chronic (slowly developing). It has many characteristic features, but it varies greatly from person to person. Its cause is unknown.

Defecation/defaecation: the act of passing faeces (stools).

Diarrhoea: the passage of unusually loose (unformed) stools. Not increased frequency of defecation, though often associated with it.

Diverticulitis: infection round a burst diverticulum.

Diverticulosis: the presence of diverticula.

Diverticulum: (plural – diverticula) an out-pouching or protruding pocket from the intestine.

ENS (enteric nervous system): a web of nerves embedded in the intestinal wall controlling the function of the intestine.

Faeces: (plural) the end-products of the digestive process as discharged from the anus.

Fibre/dietary fibre: the indigestible parts of plant foods, consisting mainly of cell walls.

Fissure/anal fissure: a split in the lining of the anal canal.

Flatulence: increased wind or gas; it can refer to increased belching as well as to increased flatus.

Flatus: gas from the anus.

Haemorrhoids: soft swellings which start in the anal canal and may protrude from the anus.

Ileostomy: a surgical procedure where an opening is constructed between the end of the small intestine (ileum) and the skin of the abdomen.

Incontinence: involuntary escape of stool from the anus (or of urine from the bladder).

Irritable bowel syndrome (IBS): a collection of symptoms blamed on the bowel, especially the colon, becoming irritable, that is, supersensitive.

Laxative: a product which helps to make passing stools easier and the stool softer.

Piles: see Haemorrhoids.

Polyp: a small swelling, often on a stalk, arising from the lining of the gut.

Proctitis: inflammation of the rectum.

Rectum: the last few inches of the bowel, above the anal canal.

Sigmoid: the last part of the colon, above the rectum.

Sigmoidoscopy: examination of the sigmoid by a telescope called a sigmoidoscope introduced via the anus. It may be a rigid metal instrument or a flexible fibreoptic one.

Travellers' diarrhoea: sudden, short-lived attack of diarrhoea brought on by bacteria (or viruses) in contaminated food or in drink taken abroad.

Useful addresses

The Digestive Diseases Foundation
(The Charity for Research and
Information on all Digestive Disorders)
3 St. Andrew's Place,
London NW1 4LB
Tel: (0171) 487 5332
For any information write to:
PO Box 251,
Edgeware,
Middlesex HA8 6HG

The Continence Foundation
307 Hatton Square,
16 Baldwin's Gardens,
London EC1N 7RJ
Helpline: (0171) 831 9831
(Mon–Fri 9.30 a.m.–4.30 p.m.)

IBS Network – The Irritable Bowel Syndrome Network
Tel: (01742) 6115231 (answerphone)
or (0181) 698 4611, ext. 8194 (restricted
hours)
Members receive a quarterly newsletter –
Gut Reaction – which is partly written by
sufferers of IBS. Members also receive a
'Can't Wait' card.

NACC
The National Association for
Colitis and Crohn's Disease
Tel: (01727) 844296
(Mon–Thurs 10 a.m.–1 p.m.)
Answerphone at other times.

Spinal Injuries Association (SIA)
76 St. James' Lane,
London N10 3DF
Helpline: (0181) 444 2121 for advice.
There are also counselling and 'link'
schemes to bring people together.
A factsheet is provided on bowel and
bladder management for the disabled.

Index

Acknowledgements

PUBLISHER'S ACKNOWLEDGEMENTS
Dorling Kindersley would like to thank the following for their help
and participation in this project:

Editorial: Nicola Munro; **Design:** Adam Powers; **DTP:** Rachel Symons;
Consultancy: Dr. Sue Davidson; **Indexing:** Indexing Specialists;
Administration: Christopher Gordon.

Organisations: St. John's Ambulance, St. Andrew's Ambulance
Organisation, British Red Cross.

Photography: (p.34, p.46, p.54) Paul Mattock; **Illustration:** (p.71) Philip Wilson;
Picture research: Angela Anderson; **Picture librarian:** Charlotte Oster.

PICTURE CREDITS
The publisher would like to thank the following for their kind
permission to reproduce their photographs. Every effort has been made
to trace the copyright holders. Dorling Kindersley apologises for any
unintentional omissions and would be pleased, in any such cases, to
add an acknowledgement in future editions.

Robert Harding Picture Library p.61;
Science Photo Library: Camr/A B Dowsett p.9;
CNRI p.3, p.50, p.80; **Tony Stone** p.46.